TIME
TO
CHANGE
YOUR
BODY

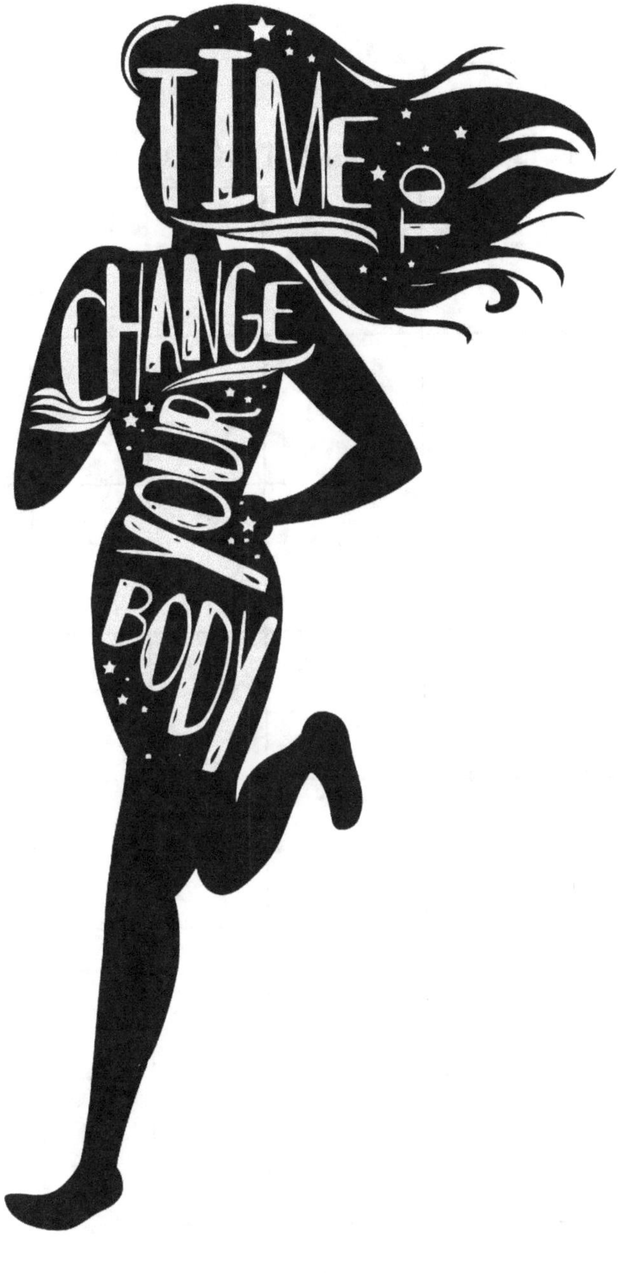

WORKOUT LOG

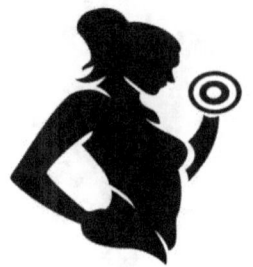

Date: _____

Weight: _____

Exercise	Weight	Reps	Sets	Notes

WORKOUT LOG

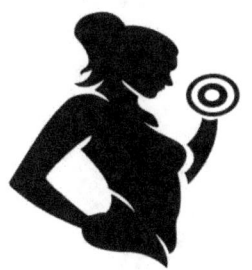

Date: _____

Weight: _____

Exercise	Weight	Reps	Sets	Notes

WORKOUT LOG

Date: _____

Weight: _____

Exercise	Weight	Reps	Sets	Notes

WORKOUT LOG

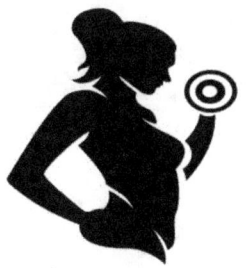

Date: _____

Weight: _____

Exercise	Weight	Reps	Sets	Notes

WORKOUT LOG

Date: _____

Weight: _____

Exercise	Weight	Reps	Sets	Notes

WORKOUT LOG

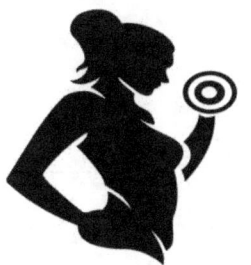

Date: _____

Weight: _____

Exercise	Weight	Reps	Sets	Notes

WORKOUT LOG

Date: _____

Weight: _____

Exercise	Weight	Reps	Sets	Notes

WORKOUT LOG

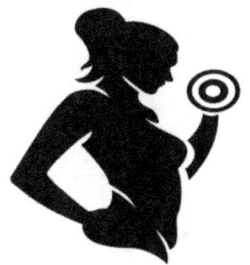

Date: _____

Weight: _____

Exercise	Weight	Reps	Sets	Notes

WORKOUT LOG

Date: _____

Weight: _____

Exercise	Weight	Reps	Sets	Notes

WORKOUT LOG

Date: _____

Weight: _____

Exercise	Weight	Reps	Sets	Notes

WORKOUT LOG

Date: _____

Weight: _____

Exercise	Weight	Reps	Sets	Notes

WORKOUT LOG

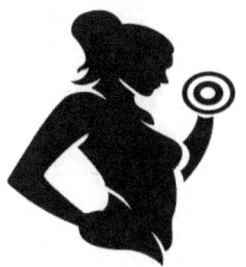

Date: _____

Weight: _____

Exercise	Weight	Reps	Sets	Notes

WORKOUT LOG

Date: _____

Weight: _____

Exercise	Weight	Reps	Sets	Notes

WORKOUT LOG

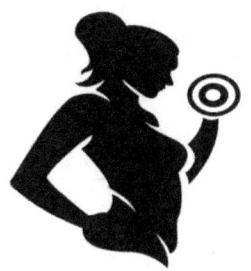

Date: _____

Weight: _____

Exercise	Weight	Reps	Sets	Notes

WORKOUT LOG

Date: _____

Weight: _____

Exercise	Weight	Reps	Sets	Notes

WORKOUT LOG

Date: _____

Weight: _____

Exercise	Weight	Reps	Sets	Notes

WORKOUT LOG

Date: _____

Weight: _____

Exercise	Weight	Reps	Sets	Notes

WORKOUT LOG

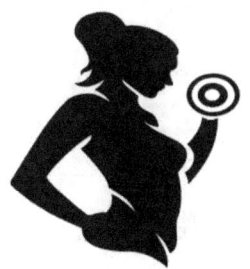

Date: _____

Weight: _____

Exercise	Weight	Reps	Sets	Notes

WORKOUT LOG

Date: _____

Weight: _____

Exercise	Weight	Reps	Sets	Notes

WORKOUT LOG

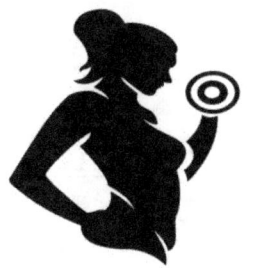

Date: _____

Weight: _____

Exercise	Weight	Reps	Sets	Notes

WORKOUT LOG

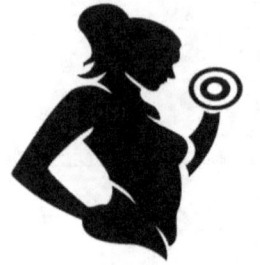

Date: _____

Weight: _____

Exercise	Weight	Reps	Sets	Notes

WORKOUT LOG

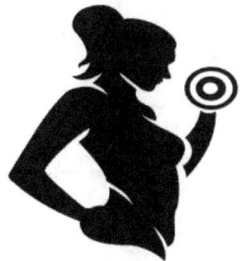

Date: _____

Weight: _____

Exercise	Weight	Reps	Sets	Notes

WORKOUT LOG

Date: _____

Weight: _____

Exercise	Weight	Reps	Sets	Notes

WORKOUT LOG

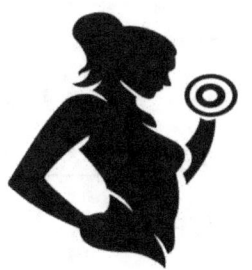

Date: _____

Weight: _____

Exercise	Weight	Reps	Sets	Notes

WORKOUT LOG

Date: _____

Weight: _____

Exercise	Weight	Reps	Sets	Notes

WORKOUT LOG

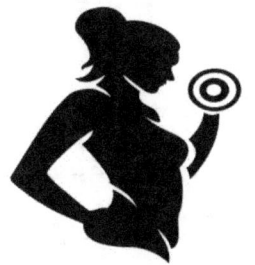

Date: _____

Weight: _____

Exercise	Weight	Reps	Sets	Notes

WORKOUT LOG

Date: _____

Weight: _____

Exercise	Weight	Reps	Sets	Notes

WORKOUT LOG

Date: _____

Weight: _____

Exercise	Weight	Reps	Sets	Notes

WORKOUT LOG

Date: _____

Weight: _____

Exercise	Weight	Reps	Sets	Notes

WORKOUT LOG

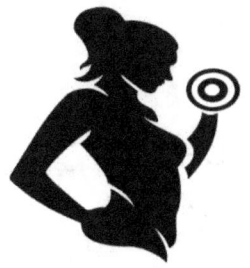

Date: _____

Weight: _____

Exercise	Weight	Reps	Sets	Notes

WORKOUT LOG

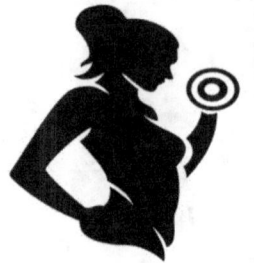

Date: _____

Weight: _____

Exercise	Weight	Reps	Sets	Notes

WORKOUT LOG

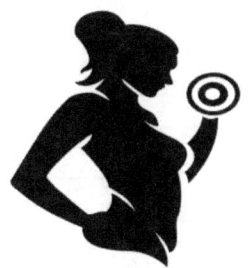

Date: _____

Weight: _____

Exercise	Weight	Reps	Sets	Notes

WORKOUT LOG

Date: _____

Weight: _____

Exercise	Weight	Reps	Sets	Notes

WORKOUT LOG

Date: _____

Weight: _____

Exercise	Weight	Reps	Sets	Notes

WORKOUT LOG

Date: _____

Weight: _____

Exercise	Weight	Reps	Sets	Notes

WORKOUT LOG

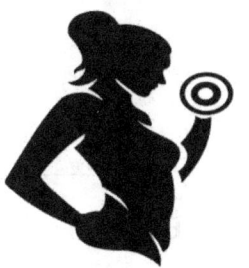

Date: _____

Weight: _____

Exercise	Weight	Reps	Sets	Notes

WORKOUT LOG

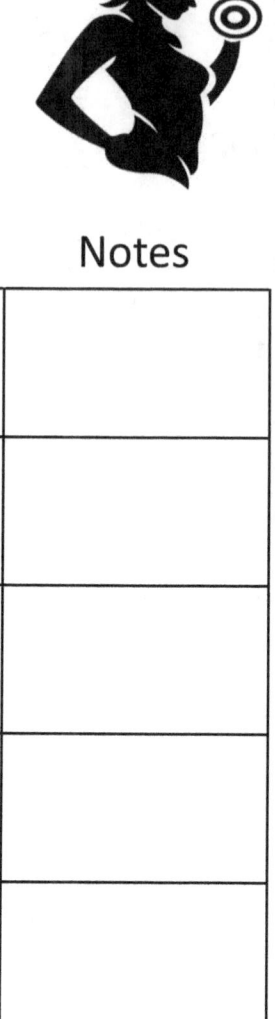

Date: _____

Weight: _____

Exercise	Weight	Reps	Sets	Notes

WORKOUT LOG

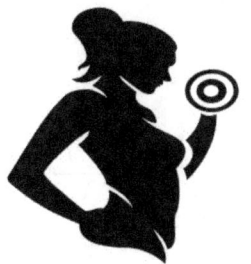

Date: _____

Weight: _____

Exercise	Weight	Reps	Sets	Notes

WORKOUT LOG

Date: _____

Weight: _____

Exercise	Weight	Reps	Sets	Notes

WORKOUT LOG

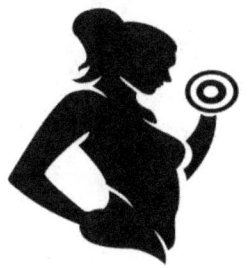

Date: _____

Weight: _____

Exercise	Weight	Reps	Sets	Notes

WORKOUT LOG

Date: _____

Weight: _____

Exercise	Weight	Reps	Sets	Notes

WORKOUT LOG

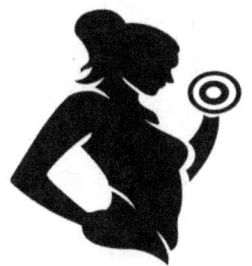

Date: _____

Weight: _____

Exercise	Weight	Reps	Sets	Notes

WORKOUT LOG

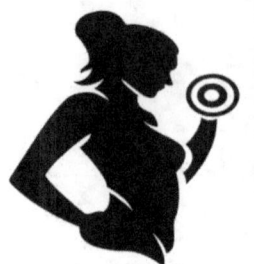

Date: _____

Weight: _____

Exercise	Weight	Reps	Sets	Notes

WORKOUT LOG

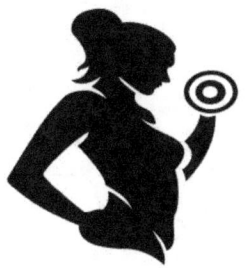

Date: _____

Weight: _____

Exercise	Weight	Reps	Sets	Notes

WORKOUT LOG

Date: _____

Weight: _____

Exercise	Weight	Reps	Sets	Notes

WORKOUT LOG

Date: _____

Weight: _____

Exercise	Weight	Reps	Sets	Notes

WORKOUT LOG

Date: _____

Weight: _____

Exercise	Weight	Reps	Sets	Notes

WORKOUT LOG

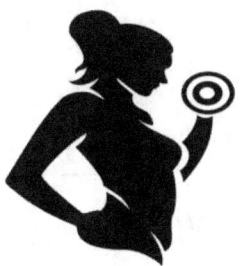

Date: _____

Weight: _____

Exercise	Weight	Reps	Sets	Notes

WORKOUT LOG

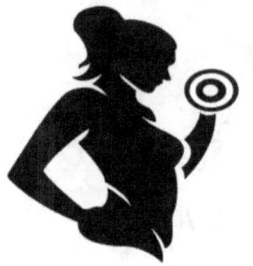

Date: _____

Weight: _____

Exercise	Weight	Reps	Sets	Notes

WORKOUT LOG

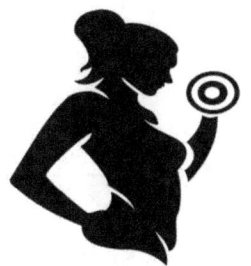

Date: _____

Weight: _____

Exercise	Weight	Reps	Sets	Notes

WORKOUT LOG

Date: _____

Weight: _____

Exercise	Weight	Reps	Sets	Notes

WORKOUT LOG

Date: _____

Weight: _____

Exercise	Weight	Reps	Sets	Notes

WORKOUT LOG

Date: _____

Weight: _____

Exercise	Weight	Reps	Sets	Notes

WORKOUT LOG

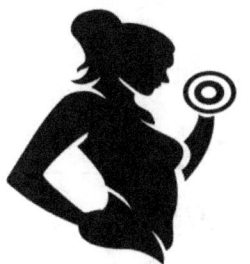

Date: _____

Weight: _____

Exercise	Weight	Reps	Sets	Notes

WORKOUT LOG

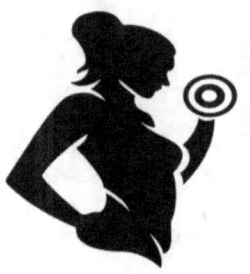

Date: _____

Weight: _____

Exercise	Weight	Reps	Sets	Notes

WORKOUT LOG

Date: _____

Weight: _____

Exercise	Weight	Reps	Sets	Notes

WORKOUT LOG

Date: _____

Weight: _____

Exercise	Weight	Reps	Sets	Notes

WORKOUT LOG

Date: _____

Weight: _____

Exercise	Weight	Reps	Sets	Notes

WORKOUT LOG

Date: _____

Weight: _____

Exercise	Weight	Reps	Sets	Notes

WORKOUT LOG

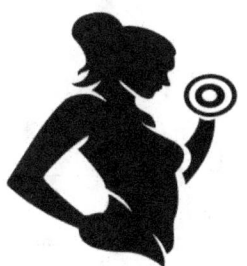

Date: _____

Weight: _____

Exercise	Weight	Reps	Sets	Notes

WORKOUT LOG

Date: _____

Weight: _____

Exercise	Weight	Reps	Sets	Notes

WORKOUT LOG

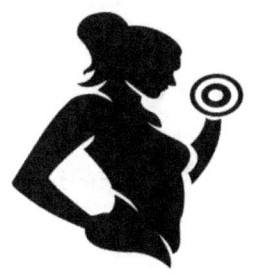

Date: _____

Weight: _____

Exercise	Weight	Reps	Sets	Notes

WORKOUT LOG

Date: _____

Weight: _____

Exercise	Weight	Reps	Sets	Notes

WORKOUT LOG

Date: _____

Weight: _____

Exercise	Weight	Reps	Sets	Notes

WORKOUT LOG

Date: _____

Weight: _____

Exercise	Weight	Reps	Sets	Notes

WORKOUT LOG

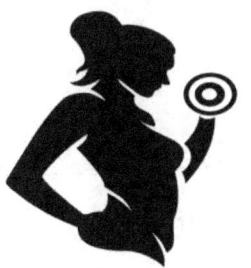

Date: _____

Weight: _____

Exercise	Weight	Reps	Sets	Notes

WORKOUT LOG

Date: _____

Weight: _____

Exercise	Weight	Reps	Sets	Notes

WORKOUT LOG

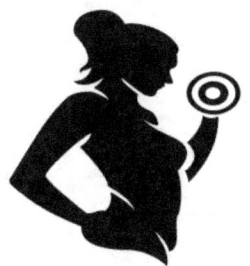

Date: _____

Weight: _____

Exercise	Weight	Reps	Sets	Notes

WORKOUT LOG

Date: _____

Weight: _____

Exercise	Weight	Reps	Sets	Notes

WORKOUT LOG

Date: _____

Weight: _____

Exercise	Weight	Reps	Sets	Notes

WORKOUT LOG

Date: _____

Weight: _____

Exercise	Weight	Reps	Sets	Notes

WORKOUT LOG

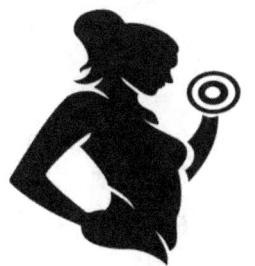

Date: _____

Weight: _____

Exercise	Weight	Reps	Sets	Notes

WORKOUT LOG

Date: _____

Weight: _____

Exercise	Weight	Reps	Sets	Notes

WORKOUT LOG

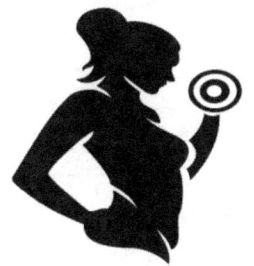

Date: _____

Weight: _____

Exercise	Weight	Reps	Sets	Notes

WORKOUT LOG

Date: _____

Weight: _____

Exercise	Weight	Reps	Sets	Notes

WORKOUT LOG

Date: _____

Weight: _____

Exercise	Weight	Reps	Sets	Notes

WORKOUT LOG

Date: _____

Weight: _____

Exercise	Weight	Reps	Sets	Notes

WORKOUT LOG

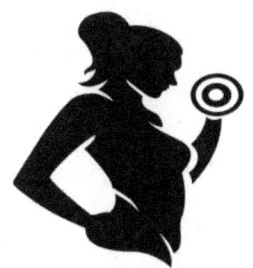

Date: _____

Weight: _____

Exercise	Weight	Reps	Sets	Notes

WORKOUT LOG

Date: _____

Weight: _____

Exercise	Weight	Reps	Sets	Notes

WORKOUT LOG

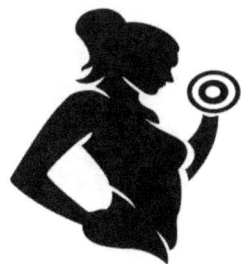

Date: _____

Weight: _____

Exercise	Weight	Reps	Sets	Notes

WORKOUT LOG

Date: _____

Weight: _____

Exercise	Weight	Reps	Sets	Notes

WORKOUT LOG

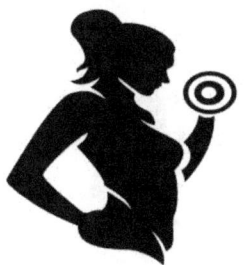

Date: _____

Weight: _____

Exercise	Weight	Reps	Sets	Notes

WORKOUT LOG

Date: _____

Weight: _____

Exercise	Weight	Reps	Sets	Notes

WORKOUT LOG

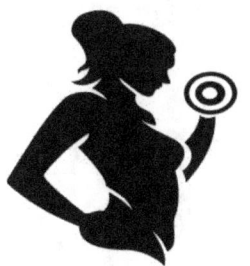

Date: _____

Weight: _____

Exercise	Weight	Reps	Sets	Notes

WORKOUT LOG

Date: _____

Weight: _____

Exercise	Weight	Reps	Sets	Notes

WORKOUT LOG

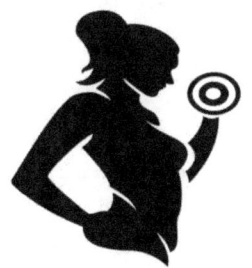

Date: _____

Weight: _____

Exercise	Weight	Reps	Sets	Notes

WORKOUT LOG

Date: _____

Weight: _____

Exercise	Weight	Reps	Sets	Notes

WORKOUT LOG

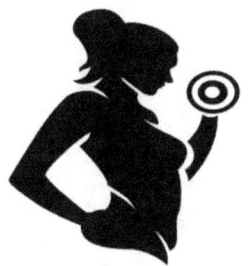

Date: _____

Weight: _____

Exercise	Weight	Reps	Sets	Notes

WORKOUT LOG

Date: _____

Weight: _____

Exercise	Weight	Reps	Sets	Notes

WORKOUT LOG

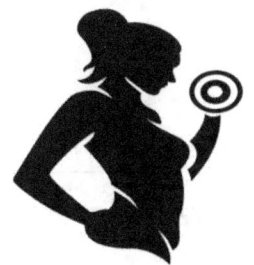

Date: _____

Weight: _____

Exercise	Weight	Reps	Sets	Notes

WORKOUT LOG

Date: _____

Weight: _____

Exercise	Weight	Reps	Sets	Notes

WORKOUT LOG

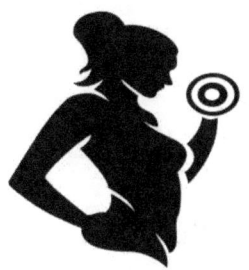

Date: _____

Weight: _____

Exercise	Weight	Reps	Sets	Notes

WORKOUT LOG

Date: _____

Weight: _____

Exercise	Weight	Reps	Sets	Notes

WORKOUT LOG

Date: _____

Weight: _____

Exercise	Weight	Reps	Sets	Notes

WORKOUT LOG

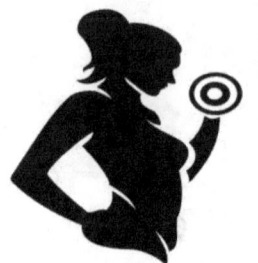

Date: _____

Weight: _____

Exercise	Weight	Reps	Sets	Notes

WORKOUT LOG

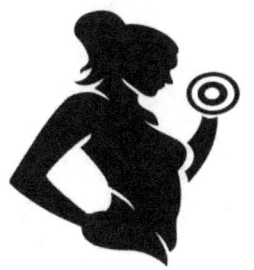

Date: _____

Weight: _____

Exercise	Weight	Reps	Sets	Notes

WORKOUT LOG

Date: _____

Weight: _____

Exercise	Weight	Reps	Sets	Notes

WORKOUT LOG

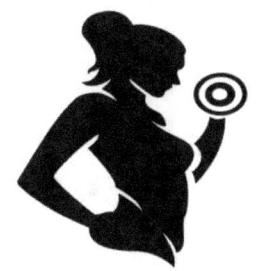

Date: _____

Weight: _____

Exercise	Weight	Reps	Sets	Notes

WORKOUT LOG

Date: _____

Weight: _____

Exercise	Weight	Reps	Sets	Notes

WORKOUT LOG

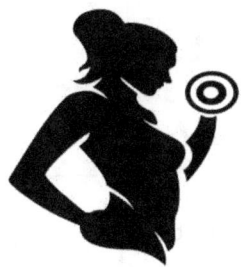

Date: _____

Weight: _____

Exercise	Weight	Reps	Sets	Notes

WORKOUT LOG

Date: _____

Weight: _____

Exercise	Weight	Reps	Sets	Notes

WORKOUT LOG

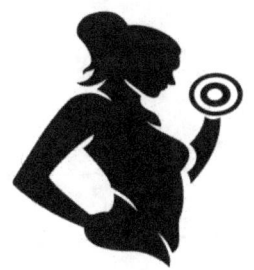

Date: _____

Weight: _____

Exercise	Weight	Reps	Sets	Notes

WORKOUT LOG

Date: _____

Weight: _____

Exercise	Weight	Reps	Sets	Notes

WORKOUT LOG

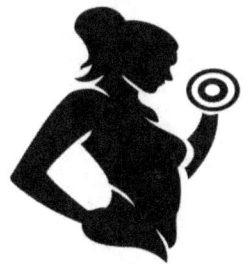

Date: _____

Weight: _____

Exercise	Weight	Reps	Sets	Notes

WORKOUT LOG

Date: _____

Weight: _____

Exercise	Weight	Reps	Sets	Notes

WORKOUT LOG

Date: _____

Weight: _____

Exercise	Weight	Reps	Sets	Notes

WORKOUT LOG

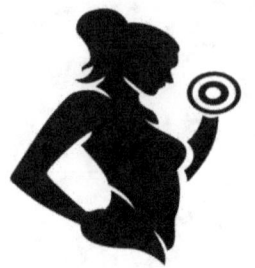

Date: _____

Weight: _____

Exercise	Weight	Reps	Sets	Notes

WORKOUT LOG

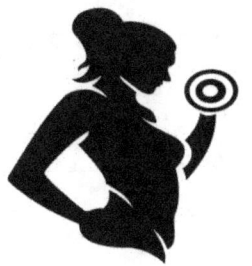

Date: _____

Weight: _____

Exercise	Weight	Reps	Sets	Notes

WORKOUT LOG

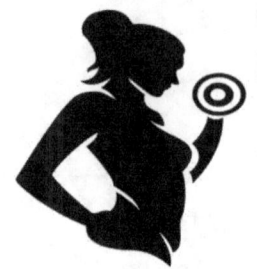

Date: _____

Weight: _____

Exercise	Weight	Reps	Sets	Notes

WORKOUT LOG

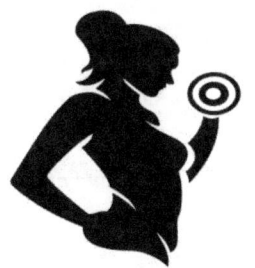

Date: _____

Weight: _____

Exercise	Weight	Reps	Sets	Notes

WORKOUT LOG

Date: _____

Weight: _____

Exercise	Weight	Reps	Sets	Notes

WORKOUT LOG

Date: _____

Weight: _____

Exercise	Weight	Reps	Sets	Notes

WORKOUT LOG

Date: _____

Weight: _____

Exercise	Weight	Reps	Sets	Notes

WORKOUT LOG

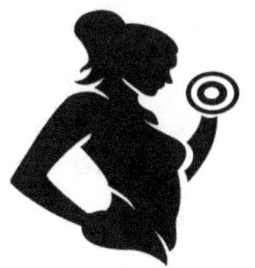

Date: _____

Weight: _____

Exercise	Weight	Reps	Sets	Notes

WORKOUT LOG

Date: _____

Weight: _____

Exercise	Weight	Reps	Sets	Notes

WORKOUT LOG

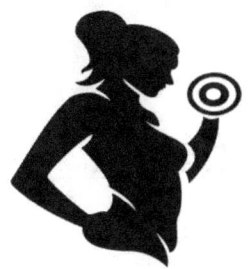

Date: _____

Weight: _____

Exercise	Weight	Reps	Sets	Notes

WORKOUT LOG

Date: _____

Weight: _____

Exercise	Weight	Reps	Sets	Notes

WORKOUT LOG

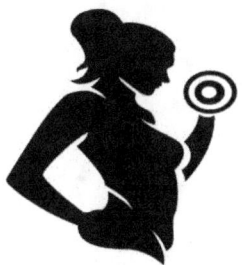

Date: _____

Weight: _____

Exercise	Weight	Reps	Sets	Notes

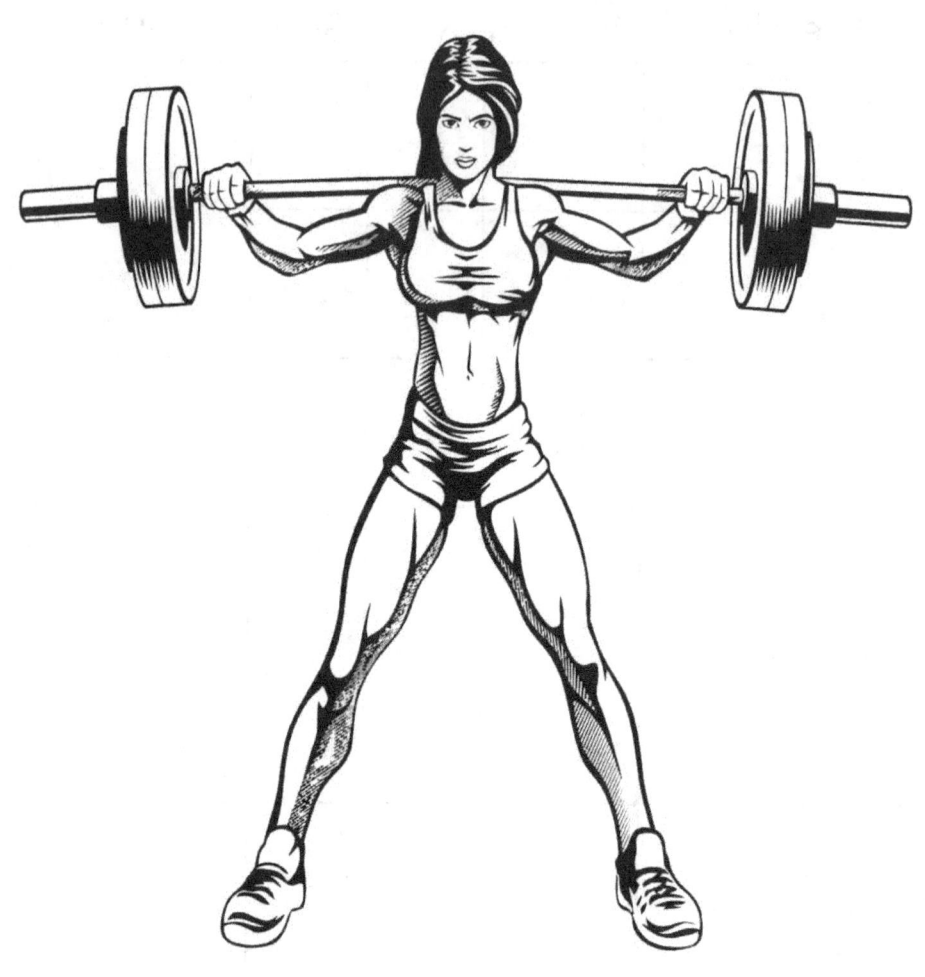